GET YOUR DREAM BODY

Build, Shape and Tone in Your Own Home

ANDREW STONE

Table of Content

Introduction

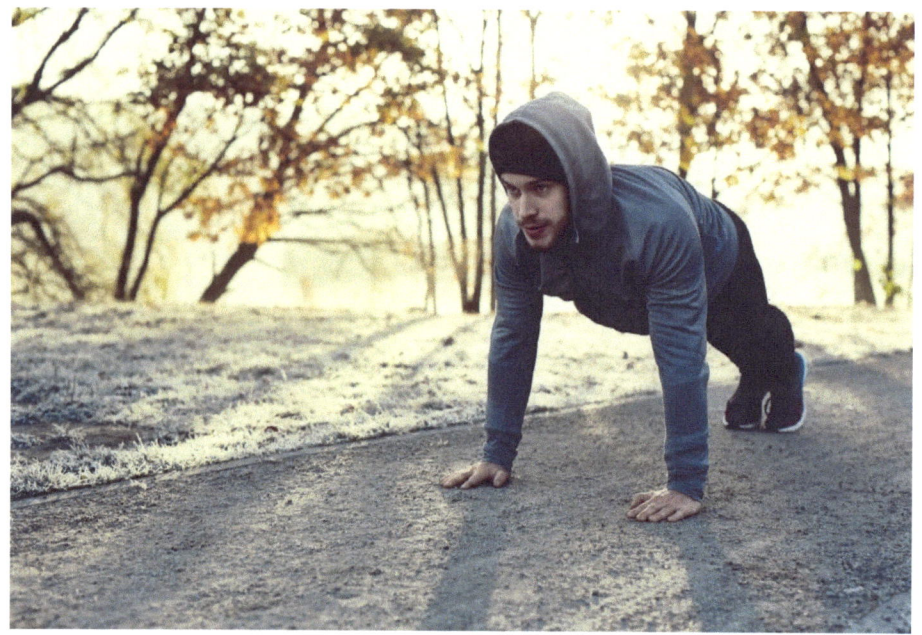

Hello there! Three cheers for downloading the book

"GET YOUR DREAM BODY

Build, Shape and Tone in Your Own Home"!

You have definitely taken a very significant step towards learning Bodyweight Exercises. What you are going to learn in this training guide is how to effectively master the basics of bodyweight workouts which do not require free-weights at all!

The book contains well-established and verified strategies as well as effective steps on how to successfully incorporate bodyweight exercises into your daily workout routine so that you can efficiently attain superior physical ability and a grand flattering ripped body!

As bodyweight workouts do not need free-weights, these are the perfect option for those who, though very much concerned about being fit, don't have access to any gym or weights. In the case of bodyweight exercises, you own weight offers the much-required resistance for the movement. For instance, push-ups, sit-ups, pull-ups, and squats are some of most frequently performed bodyweight workouts. In addition, general household items (such as a chair, sofa or towel) can also be utilized or improvised as a substitute for gym equipment.

As compared to gym workouts, which involve heavy weights and machines, bodyweight workouts have lesser injury-risks thanks to the lack of heavy load which can put unnecessary strain on your muscles. Bodyweight workouts also come with the distinct benefit of having least bulking and weight-cutting obligations which are usually associated with weights & machines training. As a result of bulking, extra fats are accumulated in your body which further reduces your overall efficiency. Therefore, bodyweight workouts can immensely assist you in maintaining a low body fat proportion, everlastingly.

Bodyweight workouts instantly work on numerous muscle groups in your body, because of the need of large muscle groups to correctly execute a movement. For instance, when you're performing push-ups, your body needs to acquire a firm straight line, and your elbow-joints need to move from 180-degree angle to the least possible angle. Here, your triceps, chest-muscles, legs, and core muscles all work simultaneously to make sure that your body acquires an appropriate and firm shape.

Many individuals believe that bodyweight exercises never truly help to improve your weightlifting capability. Their concern could be somewhat true as such exercises utilize your own weight to offer the resistance, and the weight you actually lift is not heavier than your own weight. As a result, it could be real hard for you to attain a level of intensity which is much needed for strength training. You can enhance the intensity of your bodyweight workouts by using extra weights while performing exercises such as sit-ups; however, the use of weights will go against its universal principle that the exercises should only utilize the body-weight to offer the resistance.

Nevertheless, the level of intensity can be effectively enhanced without using any weights, but by varying the leverage. You need to put more stress on particular muscle groups or limbs. For instance, you can perform one-legged squat that is way more powerful than a two-legged one. Likewise, you can perform various other exercises such as one-hand push-ups, one-hand pull-ups, and much more! Intensity levels can also be enhanced by incorporating explosiveness, or escalating volume of your movements, or even slowing-it-down to enhance the pressure on the designated muscles. These are some of the perfect ways to enhance the intensity level of your bodyweight exercises.

For some starters, a gym can be an extremely daunting experience! The bodyweight exercises can provide you with immense psychological benefit apart from other evident advantages such as convenience and economic. Bear in mind that bodyweight exercises are a great choice only if they encourage you to incorporate them as a regular habit.

Even if in due course you wish to perform weight training, a bodyweight workout is a great way to begin, and eventually perhaps the best approach. Bodyweight training can immensely help you to achieve more than what you actually imagined initially. These are exceedingly joint-friendly and permits you to perform more natural body movements. These exercises will educate you on how to effectively make use of full body strain, which is a must for learning the ways to properly manage heavy gym weights.

Once you go through this whole book, you'll come to know how easy it was to learn bodyweight exercises! In this book, I have clarified layer-by-layer all the air of secrecy surrounding bodyweight training, so that you all can readily grasp everything smoothly, fairly and speedily!

So, without further ado, LET'S GET STARTED!

Chapter 1: Bodyweight Exercise Equipment

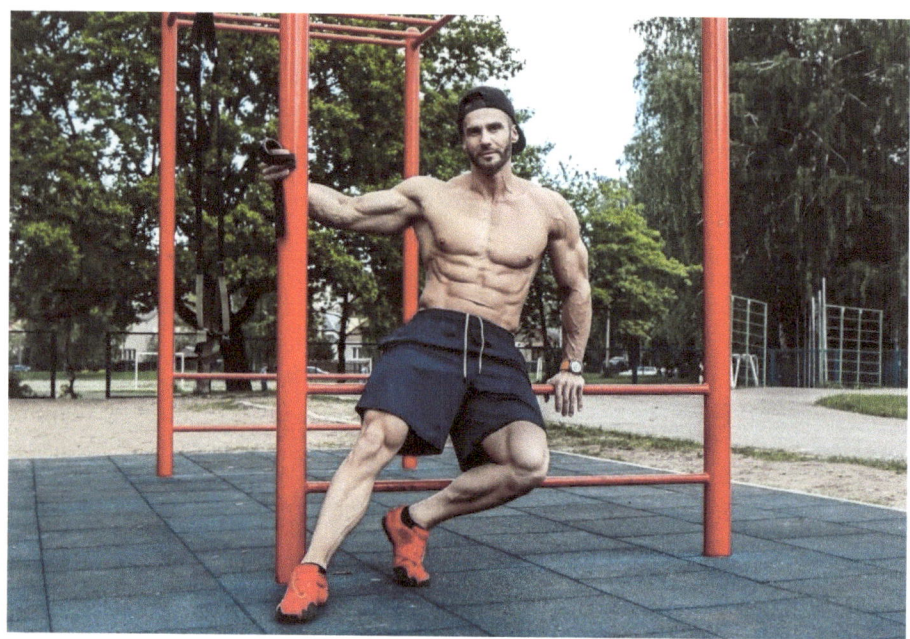

Please don't get confused or discouraged by the title of this chapter. Of course, bodyweight exercises can be performed without any free weights or gym equipment! However, our main motive or concern is to attain the maximum benefits from these workouts, and bodyweight exercise equipment will certainly help you to achieve the best results.

Bodyweight exercises are all about the fundamentals, and the fact is, no matter how much expertise you've gained in strength training, your body will, at all times, rely upon its base-level strength. Simply put, your base-level bodyweight strength will always serve as the platform as well as a link to your other strengths.

In reality, many beginners and trainees often tend to pass over and sometimes even overlook these vital bodyweight exercises. Nonetheless, you can surely gain the desired well-sculpted body as well as amazing strength when you opt to regularly perform the bodyweight workouts.

Following are some of the factors which you should keep in mind while choosing bodyweight exercise equipment:

1.1) Workout Locations:

One of the best benefits of opting for bodyweight workout is that you can perform it anywhere! You can exercise in your bedroom, your living room, at a park, or even at a gym. The only prerequisite is that the locations must be a little bit spacious to fully allow free-flow body movements. That's it!

You can even purchase various bodyweight exercise equipment and install it at your home. In addition, you can even search for any open street workout locations near your residence. These street workout locations include monkey bars, horizontal bars, chin-up bars, pull-up bars, and even Swedish Wall to train for bodyweight workouts. These components are attached together to allow you to sway around.

1.2) Proper Workout Clothing:

Your exercise attire must be more about your comfort and overall fit, and not just about making style statement only. Your workout attire can directly impact the success of the bodyweight exercises you're performing. Therefore, you need to choose proper workout clothing which makes you feel comfortable and also fits well. Following are some of the top tips to choose the perfect bodyweight workout attire:

- You need to avoid cotton fabric clothes as they absorb the sweat quickly, and don't allow it to evaporate speedily. Certainly, that's the reason why cotton attires sometimes feel wet and heavy during workouts.

- If you perspire a lot, then you should opt for the clothes with wicking ability in order to keep you dry and comfy. You can choose a Lycra/polyester blend or any other synthetic fabric to keep you cool during the summers and warm during the winters, and when you perspire, it even dries up quickly!

- Your exercise clothing must be layer-able and versatile to maintain your body temperature during the hottest as well as the coldest months. To avail the best deals, you can buy them during off-seasons. Choose a wetness-wicking dry layer, for instance, a wicking tank or T-shirt. You can even add a warmer layer like a fleece cardigan during winters.

- You can also opt for some of the modern day workout attires that come with anti-microbial cures to counter odor.

- Ensure that you choose the right workout clothing which makes you feel comfortable while performing the workout activities. Simply try it out before purchasing.

- Opt for appropriate shoes. Ensure that you wear comfy sports shoes which can efficiently support your ankles and feet.

1.3) Pull up bar:

The pull-up bar is considered as one of the most valuable and adjustable bodyweight exercise equipment. It utilizes your own weight to instantly work on numerous muscle groups in your body, and to attain this level of intensity is almost impossible with any other standard gym equipment.

When you perform bodyweight exercises on a pull-up bar, your entire body is hanging freely, which means that each of the body movements works on your core muscles with the aim of stabilizing your body. The combination of frequent extension and flexion body movements with static muscle contractions impacts various muscle groups from every angle. In a nutshell, with pull up bar you can perform nearly anything!

Following are some of the powerful bodyweight exercises which you can perform with a pull-up bar:

- Simple Pull ups
- Chin ups
- Burpee Pull ups
- Knees to elbows (cross fit)
- Hanging Knee raises
- Hanging Leg raises
- Hanging L-sits
- Muscle ups
- Windshield Wipers

1.4) Dip bars:

Dip bars are a vital part of bodyweight workout equipment which must be put into use for a number of reasons. It can be effectively utilized for more than just performing dips only. Even though you can exercise on dip bars available at any local gym, there are several lightweight versions which you can easily buy and install at your home. You can even purchase a combo of dip and pull up station as single piece exercise equipment.

The best thing about dip bars is that nothing much can go erroneous with them. And although, dip bars might come with a very basic design, these essentially offer loads of benefits to the users. Bodyweight workouts using dip bars effectively work the pectorals, back, triceps, shoulder, and Latissimi dorsi (lats) muscles simultaneously. Possibly that's the reason why all gyms have dip bars.

Following are some of the powerful bodyweight exercises which you can perform with a dip bar:

- Simple dips
- Leg raises
- Chest dips
- Modified pull-ups
- Modified push-ups (you can even perform push-ups without using dip bar).
- Weighted dips

1.5) Foam roller:

Foam rollers are reasonably priced and an extremely adaptable piece of bodyweight exercise equipment which can certainly assist you with everything, right from working out the joints in your muscle groups to carving an amazing set of core muscles faster! Simply put, if you aren't using it by now, then you're surely missing out some great workout benefits!

Also renowned as 'Self-myofascial release', foam rolling bodyweight exercises apply pressure on certain parts of your body in order to ease out pain. Performing foam rolling bodyweight exercises is effectively a more reasonable approach to offer your overall body a deep tissue rubdown. By leisurely rolling over various parts of your body, it'll assist you in breaking up scar tissues as well as adhesions, and pace up the curing and revival process during your post-workout session.

Recent research has revealed that foam rolling workouts considerably boosts the range of body movements, and also the combo of foam rolling and static stretching exercises results in maximum flexibility progress.

You can do foam rolling bodyweight workouts separately, or you can even merge them as a short ten-minute post or pre-workout session. It is recommended that the foam rolling workouts must be done once your muscles get warm. Therefore, you'll have to perform a swift 5-minute warm-up if you wish to do foam roller workouts prior to your rigorous bodyweight training session.

To perform each foam rolling workout routine, you first need to slowly roll backward and forward for about 30 seconds and then begin the next routine. While rolling, you need to take slow and deep breaths to allow your muscles to unwind. Never roll onto your joints! The foam roller must always be rolled under your muscles only, and while rolling if you feel pain at a precise stiff or soft spot, simply halt rolling and put direct pressure on that spot for about half a minute, or till the soreness reduces.

If you're just a beginner and know nothing about foam rolling exercises, just incorporate the following foam rolling moves into your daily bodyweight training routine once or twice on a daily basis, both prior to and straight away after finishing your training session.

Following are some of the powerful bodyweight exercises which you can perform with a foam roller:

- Upper back roll
- Lower back roll
- Calf roll
- Groin roll
- IT Band roll
- Hamstrings roll
- Quadriceps roll
- Lats roll
- Glutes roll
- Chest roll

1.6) Parallettes:

You don't need to become a gymnast in order to achieve all the benefits of the strength training which you can attain with parallettes. In reality, you don't even have to join any gymnastics coaching center! You just need to buy a pair of little parallette bars and begin your bodyweight workouts at home. A pair of wooden parallette bars would cost you about 50 bucks. And although aluminum parallette bars cost a bit more, you can even create a much cheaper version using a PVC pipe.

The chief advantage of using parallette bars to perform your bodyweight exercises is that your entire body remains elevated in the air (off the ground), which in turn permits you to perform a deeper range of free-flow body movements. Parallettes are amazing bodyweight training equipment which helps you to develop your core muscles as well as upper body strength. And, if you haven't utilized these bars earlier, then surely you're missing out its huge benefits.

Parallette bars are a plain piece of tools which consumes very little space and certainly offers you with huge flexibility in your routine bodyweight workouts. You can effortlessly incorporate them into your daily workout sessions.

Parallette bars help to develop exceptional upper body stamina, which includes frontward and upright pressing power, and the better coordination of your arms, core muscles, and shoulders for superior body control. This, in turn, helps to immensely perk-up your expertise in a variety of hand balancing moves, for instance, the planche position (in gymnastics) and handstand.

Following are some of the powerful bodyweight exercises which you can perform with parallettes:

- Dips
- Push ups
- L-sits / Tuck holds
- Tuck planche
- Handstand Push-ups

Note: Both pushups and handstand pushups can be done without parallettes also.

1.7) Rings:

There are only a few workout devices that actually can help to develop a ripped and strong body as powerfully as the rings (or gymnastics rings). Many gyms have evidently started to utilize rings as a potent tool for bodyweight exercises.

Still many individuals wrongly assume that the rings are only meant for athletes who compete in sports such as gymnastics. In fact, anybody can utilize the rings to perform bodyweight exercises and attain huge benefits! The rings assist in developing overall coordination, stability, stamina, and strength, simultaneously, like no other gym equipment. Furthermore, these are pretty much affordable and easy to install.

We've all witnessed the gymnastics events during the Olympics, and we all are aware of how much stamina the rings event need. What usually people don't know about the rings, however, is how efficiently these could be utilized to develop unbelievable muscular mass and dimension.

Of course, performing bodyweight exercises using the rings aren't that easy, but it's surely worth trying. When you do workouts using the rings, you'll certainly feel a big difference!

For instance, if you perform a bodyweight workout on a pull-up bar, you'll notice that your body is the only moving thing, and all you need to do is pull your body upwards to touch the bar. However, if you do the similar workout with the rings, you can no more depend on the stability of a pull-up bar. Here, you need to stabilize the rings and simultaneously pull up your body upwards to touch the rings. The entire process necessitates more focus, strain, control, and a huge amount of effort.

Focus is the key to success here. You simply can't just perform bodyweight workouts on the rings and simultaneously allow your mind to drift while you do the repetitions. Proper coordination between mind and muscle is really essential and extremely necessary to change your overall physical build, and while performing ring workouts, you just can't afford to lose your concentration. Straight away, you'll feel better muscular tension and contraction, the moment you start working out with the rings.

Following are some of the powerful bodyweight exercises which you can perform with the rings:

- Ring pull ups
- Ring push ups
- Ring dips
- Ring handstand push-ups
- Ring muscle up
- Ring L-sit

Note: All the bodyweight workouts mentioned above can also be performed without rings.

****

In the next chapter, we'll discuss proper nutrition, rest, and recovery.

Chapter 2: Proper Nutrition, Rest, and Recovery

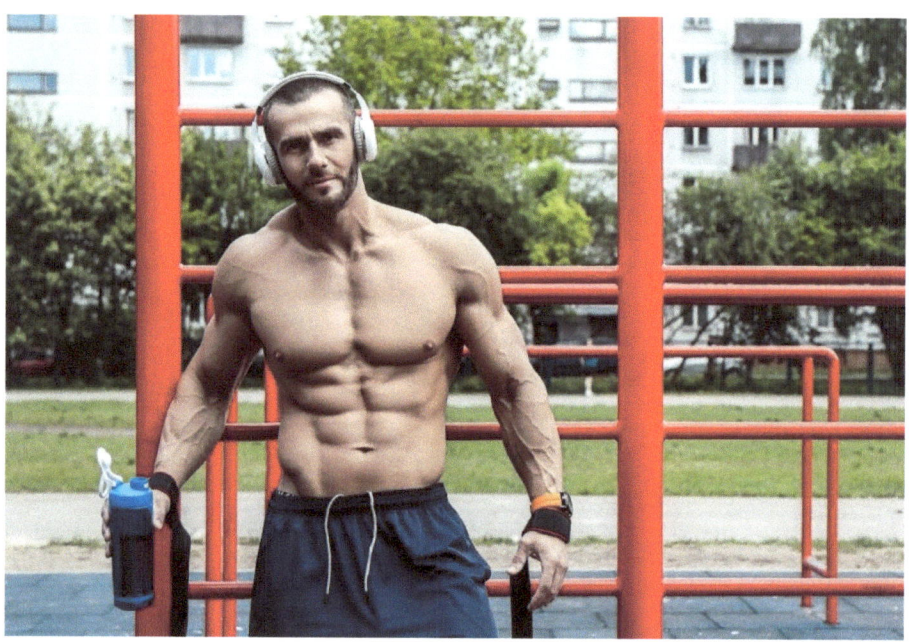

The very reason why many individuals get attracted to bodyweight exercises are their simplistic nature. You don't need to join any gym or spend money to avail the membership, and furthermore, you don't even require any gym equipment at all! Your mind and your body are all that you require, and by working them together as a team, you can perform some of the most powerful bodyweight exercises.

However, building a ripped body takes more than just hammering out these exercises. To develop a well-sculpted body, you actually need to eat right too!

If you're fully prepared to follow the proper workout nutrition and wish to make the most out of your workout efforts, then you need to take a vow to consume natural food only, and completely renounce junk food! Once you're able to make up your mind about eating right, the remaining task is pretty simple.

There are many ways to eat well and plenty of natural foods to pick from, quite similar to the various bodyweight workouts that you're able to perform. The diet isn't that complicated! You don't need to follow any intricate system, or take any supplements or pills, or purchase any expensive food items.

2.1) Consume Natural Food:

You'll never ever be able to attain lean muscles if you keep on munching burgers, french fries, soft drinks, and other junk foods. Always remember that a well-sculpted body isn't made from pastries, energy drinks, or chocolate bars. If you're damn serious about following the proper bodyweight workout diet, then you need to fully discard junk foods.

Recommended Natural Food Items:

Human beings are evolved to consume fruits and vegetables in great quantities. Such food items are fully loaded with all types of vital minerals and vitamins which your body requires not only to develop lean muscles but also to appropriately manage all the bodily functions.

Following are of some of the recommended natural food items:

- Fruits, veggies, seeds and nuts.
- Non-vegetarian food item such as meat (should be grass fed, organic)
- Steer clear of refined, sugary, starchy, and processed foods all the time.

Following is the recommended perfect meal:

- Little quantity of eggs, fish, chicken, or beef (grass fed)
- Fresh fruits (all kinds)
- Great quantity of fresh and non-starchy veggies
- Nuts, olive oil, avocado (keep away from hydrogenated oils or trans fats)

Protein Sources: The chief muscle-developing protein can be sourced from eggs, greek yogurt, beef, chicken, turkey, tuna, salmon, bison, etc.

Carbs Sources: All the vital carbs can be sourced from sprouted bread, quinoa, white potatoes, rice, sweet potatoes, fruits & veggies such as broccoli, spinach, kale, green beans, cauliflower, carrots, green peppers, eggplant, squash, etc. These food items can provide you with all the essential nutrients and power which your body requires.

Healthy Fats Sources: All the vital and healthy fatty acids which your body requires to create testosterone hormones can be sourced from almonds, avocado, nut butter, fish oil, olive oil and coconut oil.

2.2) Drink As Much Water As You Can:

Water is considered as the most vital nutrient for all the individuals who perform rigorous workouts. Consuming ample quantity of water post-workout is really necessary to replenish all the fluids which you lose during your workout session in the form of sweat. You need to maintain good hydration which in turn helps in healthy weight loss. However, if you consume extreme quantities of water post-workout, then it could lead to hyponatremia (a hazardous health condition).

Hydration:

Consuming a good amount of water post-workout helps you to replenish all the fluids which you lose during your workout session and make certain that your body remains adequately hydrated. During your rigorous workouts, your body loses a huge quantity of water in the form of sweat which could result in dehydration. Therefore, you need to replenish your body with water and other juices.

Water loss (in the form of sweat) during intense bodyweight workouts could surpass several liters. In order to check whether or not your body is sufficiently rehydrated post-workout, you need to test out your urine color. The color of your urine will be clear if you are adequately hydrated. Drinking cool water after finishing your exercise is an ideal choice. This will enable your body to restore its temperature at a normal level.

Drinking adequate water before the workout session as well as during the workouts is also very important to make sure that you're properly hydrated, particularly when you're exercising for a lengthy duration or during summers. Consuming other fluids like juice or milk can also assist in rehydrating your body post-workout.

However, you must avoid caffeinated beverages as these, in reality, promote fluid loss. Consequently, such beverages are not an ideal choice to rehydrate your body. Sports drinks (caffeine less) are a good choice specifically for those workouts which last more than an hour. Besides replenishing vital fluids in your body, sports drinks also reinstate necessary electrolytes which were lost during your rigorous bodyweight workouts.

Caution:

It is recommended to consume a good amount of water pre and post workouts. However, consuming massive gallons of water post-workout could lead to hyponatremia (a hazardous health condition), which can cause fits, unconsciousness, and even death. Hyponatremia is a rare condition among fit individuals even though it sometimes happens to sportspersons, for instance, marathon runners, who consume massive amounts of water pre and post training. The symptoms are nausea, swollen feet, and hands, confusion, fatigue, vomiting, etc.

2.3) Proper Rest and Recovery:

After finishing your intense bodyweight workouts, proper rest and recovery are crucial! Recovery period must be considered as a window of opportunity. Roughly half an hour after your rigorous workout session, your body is optimized to restore its energy stocks: both liver glycogen and muscles. The process called 'muscle-protein-synthesis' begins which initiate muscle repair and revival, replenishes much-needed fluids and helps your overall body acclimatize to the strains of the intense workout.

Proper sleep is very important for the overall growth of your muscles. You need to sleep for at least 7 to 8 hours every day. It's during your sleep only, the growth hormones are released by your body to carry out the entire muscles repair and revival task. And if you don't sleep well, you body won't release the growth hormones, and it won't go through the repair and revival cycle.

In order to sleep well, you need to make your bedroom cool and dark, and stop using PC, Smartphone or and other LED screen device, right before going to bed. Make it a habit to sleep and get up as early as possible every day to get the maximum health benefits.

****

In the next chapter, we'll talk about warming up and mobility exercises.

Chapter 3: Warming up and Mobility

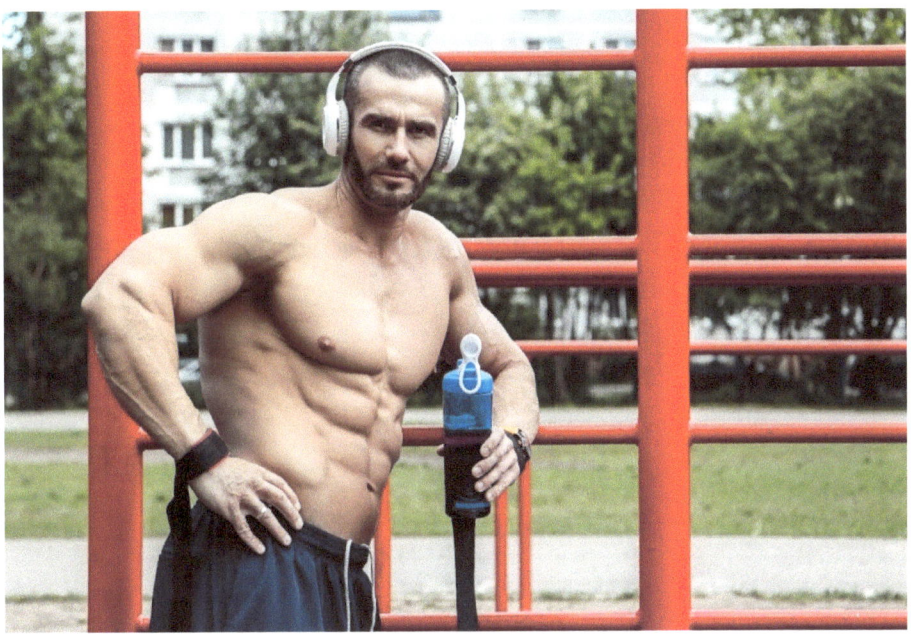

Warming up and mobility are the most misunderstood and missed out aspects of bodyweight training. Mobility is your body's capability to move freely and effortlessly, and warm-ups are the key ways to facilitate your body to accomplish this.

Humans are born with full physical mobility. However, with the aging process, we tend to lose our mobility, and gradually our bodies get stiffen up. Nevertheless, not only you can sustain your overall mobility right from an early age, you can even regain your body's capability to move effortlessly.

Proper warm ups prior to performing your bodyweight exercises will prepare your entire body by increasing its core temperature, activating the nervous system and developing joint mobility or lubrication as well as a range of body movements for maximum stamina, performance, and endurance.

The warm up and mobility exercises which we are going to discuss below contain a good combination of dynamic motions as well as various stretching exercises. These will effectively diminish all the injury risks and will allow you to perform the workouts at your best.

These warming up and mobility sessions won't take more than ten to fifteen minutes to finish. However, if you don't do these warm-up routines prior to your intense workout sessions, then there is a high chance that you might injure yourself. Bear in mind that injuries may halt your training program completely. Therefore, these mobility routines must be your primary concern at all times.

3.1) Upper Body Mobility:

Begin with 3 to 4 minutes of common cardio warm-ups such as jumping, high knee pulls, torso twists, cross-toe touches, front kicks, etc. After that, you can safely start the following upper body warm-ups and mobility exercises:

Arm Swings:

- **<u>Step 1</u>:** Attain a standing posture with your feet shoulder distance apart, and tenderly cover your chest with both of your arms as if you're hugging yourself.
- **<u>Step 2</u>:** Slowly release the arms back as if you're going to hug someone else.
- **<u>Step 3</u>:** Continue with the arm swings (hugging and releasing), as mentioned in Step 1 & 2, for about 40 to 50 seconds till you feel a bit of warm pressure in your chest and back muscles.

Arm Circles:

- **<u>Step 1</u>:** Raise and hold both of your arms parallel to the ground to your sides.
- **<u>Step 2</u>:** Rotate your arms in a little circular motion (backward circles) using your shoulder joints.
- **<u>Step 3</u>:** Slowly increase the perimeter of the circle till your arms begin to rotate in huge circles, going way above your head and way down to your knees.
- **<u>Step 4</u>:** Continue to rotate the backward circles for 30 seconds, and after that reverse the direction of the circle.
- **<u>Step 5</u>:** Again continue to rotate the forward circles for 30 seconds, and gradually increase the perimeter of the circles.

Foam Roll (Thoracic Spine):

- **Step 1:** Lie down on your back and place a foam roller behind your shoulders with your face facing the ceiling. Cover your upper body with your arms as if you're hugging yourself. This pose will separate your scapula.
- **Step 2:** Raise your hips and head to attain a neutral position, and then steadily roll over the foam up and down at the middle of your upper back 12 to 15 times.
- **Step 3:** Turn your body towards the left and do 12 to 15 foam rolls along the left side. After that, turn your body towards the right and do 12 to 15 foam rolls along the right side.

Shoulder Dislocations:

- **Step 1:** Take hold of a broomstick (or a resistance band) and begin with the broomstick or the band in front of you touching your belly.
- **Step 2:** Keep both of your arms straight and rotate them backward in a round motion all the way above your head.
- **Step 3:** Bring down the stick behind your lower back.
- **Step 4:** Perform 12 to 15 repetitions.

Note: You can have a wider or narrower grip in accordance with your shoulder flexibility and limb extent. You need to find the comfortable distance which permits a fine shoulder and arm stretch without causing any muscle pain.

3.2) Lower Body Mobility:

Begin with 3 to 4 minutes of common cardio warm-ups such as jumping jacks, torso twists, front and back kicks, toe touches, etc. After that, you can safely start the following lower body warm-ups and mobility exercises:

Cat's Arch:

- **Step 1:** Attain a kneeling position with your arms right under your shoulders, the knees right under your hips, and a neutral lower back. Breathe-in to begin, after that drop your tummy towards the ground. Bend your lower back and simultaneously curl your head upwards, and look at the roof.
- **Step 2:** Take a short pause, and then breathe out to reverse the motion. Arch your spine like a cat and simultaneously curl your head downwards and look at your belly.
- **Step 3:** Perform 12 to 15 repetitions.

Bent-Knee Iron Cross:

- **Step 1:** Lie down on your back and extend both of your arms out to your sides. Lift your legs up in the air with your thighs at right angles to the ground and your shins parallel to the ground.
- **Step 2:** Begin by simply dropping your knees to one side and simultaneously dropping your head to the opposite side.

- **Step 3:** Repeat the action by dropping your head as well as your knees the reverse way.
- **Step 4:** Perform 12 to 15 repetitions per side.

Knee Circles:

- **Step 1:** Attain a kneeling position with the hands right under your shoulders, the knees right under your hips. Raise one of your feet up to your hips.
- **Step 2:** Start sketching circles in the air with the raised knee. You need to draw as big circles as possible with the knee without changing your upper body's pose.
- **Step 3:** Perform 12 to 15 repetitions in a single direction. After that, reverse the direction. Perform the same routine with your other leg.

Leg Swings:

- **Step 1:** Attain a standing position and place your hand on a wall or any other support to gain balance. Place your entire bodyweight on your single foot and raise your other leg upwards off the floor.
- **Step 2:** Just swing the raised leg in both direction sideways or front-ways while maintaining your core muscles tight.
- **Step 3:** Perform 12 to 15 repetitions of the leg swings. After that, perform the same routine with your other leg.

3.3) Overall Body Stretching Exercises:

Forward Lunge Stretch:

- **Step 1:** Place your one foot forward and attain a lower lunge pose by positioning your fingers on the ground.
- **Step 2:** First inhale, and after that in single motion breathe out while straightening out your forward leg. Then, slowly go back to the previous lunge pose.
- **Step 3:** Perform 4 to 5 repetitions. After that, perform the entire routine with your other leg.

Side Stretches:

- **Step 1:** Attain a standing position with your feet hip's width apart and both of your arms in a straight line above your head. Hold your hands together, extend your index fingers, and take a deep breath.
- **Step 2:** Exhale and bend your entire upper body to the left side. Slowly inhale 5 breaths and return to the original position.
- **Step 3:** Perform the entire routine on the right side.

Forward Dangle:

- **Step 1:** Attain a standing position with your feet hip's width apart and bend your knees a little. Move your arms behind your back and clutch your fingers together. You can even use a broomstick or a towel. Inhale and set your arms straight to pump up your chest area.
- **Step 2:** Breathe out and bend forward, and allow your arms to stretch and move upwards from behind.
- **Step 3:** Remain in that position for 5 deep breaths. Then, return to the original position.
- **Step 4:** Perform 4 to 5 repetitions.

Forward Lunge Arch:

- **Step 1:** Place your one foot forward and attain a lower lunge position. Lower your back leg knee towards the ground. Put your arms in front of your forward leg and clip your thumbs together. The palms should face the ground.
- **Step 2:** Inhale and move your arms frontwards above your head. You need to stretch as far back as possible. Remain in that position for 5 deep breaths. Then, return to the original position.
- **Step 3:** Perform the entire routine with your other leg.

****

In the next chapter, we'll discuss various bodyweight exercises.

Chapter 4: Bodyweight Exercises

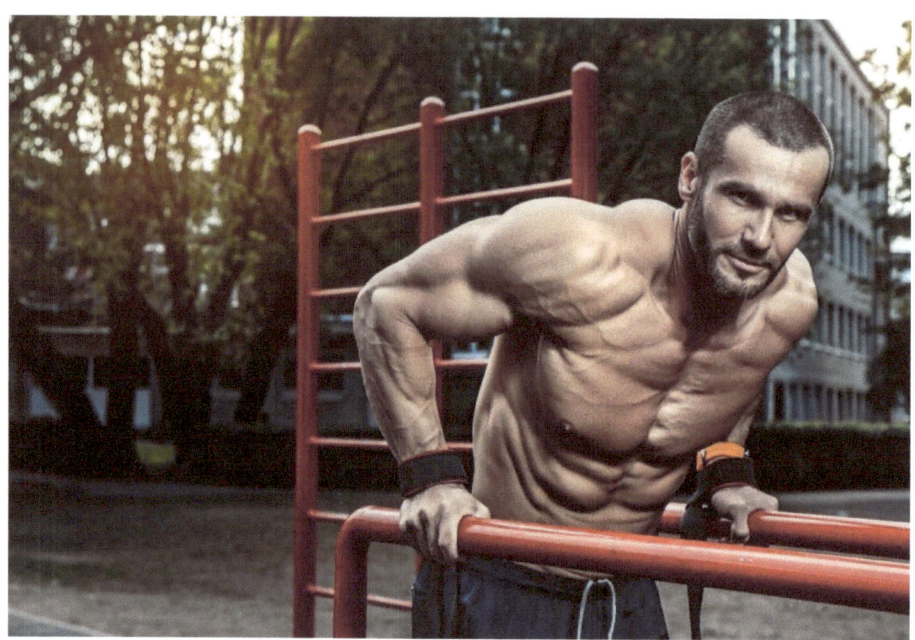

In this chapter, we'll talk about various bodyweight exercises. These exercises will cover nearly your entire body parts such as arms, neck and shoulders, core muscles, chest region, the back region, legs, thighs, calves, etc.

4.1) Bodyweight Workouts for Stronger Arms:

Your arms, quite similar to your abs, are mostly at the forefront of your mind since they appear so impressive. Everyone desires to improve the shape of their arms. Men want them huge and ripped! Women want their arms to be toned and slender!

Ripped arms are not something that you're born with! You need to put in a lot of efforts to achieve them, and the best thing about bodyweight exercises for stronger arms is that you can perform them anywhere whether you're at your home or a hotel room, a park or your backyard, your basement or bedroom – literally anywhere!

All the gym owners understand this very well, and as a result, they pack their gyms with all the latest and eye-catching equipment exclusively intended to shape up your arms. However, you don't need to join any of those fancy gyms to attain ripped arms. Just put aside all your fancy dumbbells and get ready to learn the fundamentals of bodyweight exercises. Also, if you're already using the gym equipment, by opting for bodyweight workouts you'll allow your joints as well as your entire body a much-desired break.

Achieving best results is merely a question of following a right strategy, putting in a lot of efforts, and having a positive frame of mind. By changing your body position and angle and being creative with the appropriate bodyweight training equipment, you can definitely achieve the required stimulus for the overall growth of your triceps, biceps, and forearms.

Following are some of the bodyweight exercises for stronger arms:

Diamond Push-ups:

- **Step 1:** Attain a push-up position with your index fingers and thumbs making a diamond shape on the floor.
- **Step 2:** Hold your elbows as near as possible to your sides and bring your upper body down towards the floor till your chest makes contact with your hands on the floor. During the entire motion you need to keep your core muscles, thighs, and glutes tight.
- **Step 3:** Return back to the original position.
- **Step 4:** Perform 12 to 15 repetitions.

Dips:

- **Step 1:** Balance your upper body over a dip bar (you can even use chairs or benches).
- **Step 2:** Lower down your entire body till your elbows attain a perpendicular shape.
- **Step 3:** After that, move back up to the original position by straightening out your arms. While performing the dips, you need to maintain your chest up and your back straight all through the movements.
- **Step 4:** Perform 12 to 15 repetitions.

Plank Triceps (Extensions):

- **Step 1:** Attain a plank position with your elbows right under your shoulders and your forearms straight out before you. Place your palm on the ground, and maintain your back, hips and legs straight in line.
- **Step 2:** Push your upper body up with your forearms and extend your elbows till the arms get straighten out.
- **Step 3:** Return back to the original position after 4 seconds.
- **Step 4:** Perform 12 to 15 repetitions.

Chin-ups:

- **Step 1:** Hold the pull-up bar firmly with your hands shoulder-distance apart. Tighten your core and glutes to maintain your whole body like a pillar (straight in line).
- **Step 2:** Pull your chest upwards to the bar, and drag your shoulder blades down and backward.
- **Step 3:** Halt at the top for 3 to 4 seconds and gradually lower your body down.
- **Step 4:** Perform 12 to 15 repetitions.

4.2) Bodyweight Workouts for Neck:

Most individuals are scared of performing neck exercises as they consider these might harm their necks. However, that's precisely the very reason why you should be doing the neck workouts!

The human neck has numerous muscles, and these neck muscles support the skull, cervical spine, and also the brain. Therefore these muscles have to be well-built. We'll discuss some bridging exercises. Remember, these exercises aren't just meant for your neck only. These exercises also work your spine as well as all the back muscles.

Following are some of the bodyweight exercises for a muscular neck. You need to use an exercise mat to perform these workouts:

Wrestler's Bridge Using Hands:

- **Step 1:** Lie down on the mat on your back with your knees pointing upwards and your feet flat on the mat. Place both of your hands near your head with your elbows pointing upwards.
- **Step 2:** Slowly lift your torso off the mat till your head's top is touching the mat. The hands need to stay on the mat to balance your body. Slowly lift your hips and hold the position for as long as possible.
- **Step 3:** Slowly return back to the original position.
- **Step 4:** Perform 12 to 15 repetitions.

Front Bridge Using Hands:

- **Step 1:** Attain a bear crawl position with your butts high up, and your feet and hands on the mat.
- **Step 2:** Rest your head on the mat and slowly roll your head towards the back. Keep your legs straight, and your butts high up.
- **Step 3:** Slowly roll back your head to the original position.
- **Step 4:** Perform 12 to 15 repetitions.

Neck Plank without Hands:

- **Step 1:** Attain a front bridge position and then move your feet backward. Keep your feet as close as possible. Also, keep your hands off the mat and lock it behind your back. Just your feet and your forehead must be in touch with the mat. This position is quite similar to a plank. The only difference is, instead of your hands the support is on your forehead and your neck.
- **Step 2:** Hold this position for some time, and then return back to the original pose.

4.3) Bodyweight Workouts for Shoulders:

After performing some bodyweight exercises for a while, you'll surely feel how vital it is to fortify your shoulders as these muscles are engaged in just about every motion. You simply won't be able to perform the advanced levels without strong shoulder muscle groups.

There are various bodyweight workouts specifically meant for shoulder strengthening. Furthermore, these exercises are way safer as compared to weight training programs. Many individuals sustain injuries as they don't do the workouts properly or use much bigger weights which put their shoulders under immense strain. These bodyweight exercises will certainly help you to avoid any injuries since all the movements are natural.

Following are some of the bodyweight exercises for shoulders:

Pull-ups:

- **Step 1:** Use a firm overhand grip to hold a pull-up bar with your hands a bit wider than your shoulder-distance. Keep your thighs closer and tighten your core. Your entire body needs to stay rigid for the whole movement.
- **Step 2:** Pull your entire body upwards by bringing your elbows closer to the ribs and simultaneously squeezing your shoulder blades. Let your upper chest or neck touch the pull-up bar.
- **Step 3:** Halt for some time, and then return back to the original position.
- **Step 4:** Perform 12 to 15 repetitions.

Pike Push-ups:

- **Step 1:** Attain a push-up position on the ground. Straighten out your arms with both of your hands shoulder-distance apart. Raise your hips up and allow your body to form a reverse 'V' shape. Your arms and legs need to remain straight.
- **Step 2:** Just bend your elbows only and slowly bring down your upper body to touch the ground with your head's top.
- **Step 3:** Halt for some time, and then return back to the original position.
- **Step 4:** Perform 12 to 15 repetitions.

Inverted Rows:

- **Step 1:** Use a firm overhand grip to hold the hip-height bar with your arms shoulder-distance apart. Hang with fully straightened arms and your shoulder must be right beneath your hands. Straighten your legs and keep your feet close.
- **Step 2:** Raise your chest upwards with your arms and touch the bar to your chest. Straighten your wrists all the time (don't curl them).
- **Step 3:** Halt for some time, and then return back to the original position.
- **Step 4:** Perform 12 to 15 repetitions.

Simple Push-ups:

- **Step 1:** Attain a push-up position by placing both by your hands on the ground a bit wider than your shoulder-width. Tighten your core as well as your glutes. Your toes should be touching the ground, and your ankles should be straight in line with your thighs, hips, and your back up to your head. Keep your feet close.
- **Step 2:** Lower your upper body by bending your elbows till your chest almost touches the ground.
- **Step 3:** Hold that position for some time, and then return back to the original position as fast as possible.
- **Step 4:** Perform 12 to 15 repetitions.

4.4) Bodyweight Workouts for Core Muscles:

You simply don't need to go on a hunger strike or waste hours in a gym to achieve ripped core muscles! Bodyweight workouts involve the most effective methods to strengthen as well as tone up your abs.

Your core contains various muscle groups such as lower and upper abdominals, and the glutes, psoas, back, and side muscles. It offers a muscular structure which safeguards various internal organs, helps in body movement, and provides stability and steadiness to your entire body.

Following are some of the bodyweight exercises for core muscles:

Superman Pose:

- **Step 1**: Lie down on the floor over your belly, and stretch out your legs and arms just the way Superman flies in the sky.
- **Step 2**: Raise your legs and arms up off-the-floor, and hold for 5 seconds. After that return to the original position.
- **Step 3**: Perform 20 to 25 repetitions.

Reverse Crunch Moves:

- **Step 1**: Lie down on the floor on your back. Place your hands at the sides and bend your knees. Raise your knees a little bit up off-the-floor so that your shin is parallel to the floor.
- **Step 2**: Raise your legs up using your core till your butts are also raised a bit. Remain in that position for some time and then return back to the original position. It's necessary to remain stable and not using momentum to move back-and-forth.
- **Step 3**: Perform 20 to 25 repetitions.

Mountain Climbers:

- **Step 1:** Attain a push-up position on the floor, and straighten out your arms with both of your hands shoulder-distance apart. Move your one leg forward right under your chest and stretch the other leg straight behind you.
- **Step 2:** Hold the position and then move both of your legs back-and-forth. It's quite similar to running; however, since your hands are holding firmly onto the floor, it's relatively similar to mountain climbing.

Back Bridge:

- **Step 1:** Lie down on your back on the floor. Place your heels near your hips and bend your knees. Place your arms palms-down at the sides.
- **Step 2:** Tighten your glutes and lift your butts up to attain the back bridge position. Maintain your shoulders straight in line with your back thighs and knees.
- **Step 3:** Maintain the bridge position for as long as possible and then return back to the original position.
- **Step 4:** Perform 15 to 20 repetitions.

Catapult Move:

- **Step 1:** Lie down on the floor on your back. Bend your knees and press your feet flat onto the floor. Stretch out your arms straight at the back of your head.
- **Step 2:** Beginning with your arms, shoot (catapult) your upper body upwards, and make yourself into a sitting pose.
- **Step 3:** Hold the position for a short time, and then slowly return back to the original position on the floor.
- **Step 4:** Perform 15 to 20 repetitions.

6 - Inches Lift:

- **Step 1:** Lie down on the floor on your back. Straighten out your legs, and raise them off-the-floor about 6 inches up. Hold your legs right there!
- **Step 2:** Maintain the position for 50 to 60 seconds or even more.
- **Step 3:** Perform 15 to 20 repetitions.

Boat Position:

- **Step 1:** Attain an upright seated position and straighten out your legs before you and place your arms at the sides. After that, bend your upper body backward till it almost makes 45 degrees angle with the floor.

- **Step 2**: Keep your legs closer and raise them up off-the-floor to the level of your head. Straighten out your arms right before you.
- **Step 3**: Maintain this position for as long as possible by tightening your core muscles. Then return back to the original position.
- **Step 4**: Perform 15 to 20 repetitions.

Plank:

- **Step 1**: Lie down on the floor over your belly. Push your entire body up off-the-floor on your forearms and toes. Your forearms must be in front of you. Your entire body should be straight in line from your head to toe.
- **Step 2**: Maintain this pose for as long as possible (maybe up to 5 minutes).
- **Step 3**: Perform a couple more repetitions.

Side (Transverse) Plank:

- **Step 1**: Lie down on the floor on your left side. Keep your left elbow beneath your left shoulder and your left forearm right before you for support. Place your right foot on top of your left, and place your right arm at your side.
- **Step 2**: Firmly raise your butts up off-the-floor and swing your right arm behind your head to let your body attain a straight line. After that, lower your butts down to the floor and raise it again.

- **Step 3:** Perform 10 to 15 repetitions. Then switch the sides and repeat all the steps.

Scissor Kicks:

- **Step 1:** Lie down on the floor on your back and straighten out your legs. Stretch out your arms and place your hands (palms down) beside your hips to support the back. Keep your legs close.
- **Step 2:** Lift your legs about 6 inches up off-the-floor. After that, slowly lift your shoulders up off-the-floor, and press your elbows into the floor to maintain support. Tighten up your core muscles.
- **Step 3:** Now, you have to scissor your legs by placing one leg over the other. Your right leg goes over the left leg while the left leg goes below the right leg, in the air. Again, the right leg returns and goes below the left leg while the left leg returns back and goes over the right leg. Again scissor your left leg to the right, and your right leg to the left. The entire movement needs to be done in the air.
- **Step 4:** Perform 15 to 20 repetitions.

4.5) Bodyweight Workouts for Chest:

You definitely can build an awesome chest without doing any bench presses. There are a number of great bodyweight exercises for your chest which you can perform without any fancy gym equipment. And although these workouts are great for building your chest, these will even help to work your core area, triceps, deltoids and various other upper body muscles.

Following are some of the bodyweight exercises for chest:

Side Push-ups:

- **Step 1:** Attain the usual push-up position. Straighten out your back and place your palms on the floor shoulder-distance apart. Transfer your upper body weight over one of the arms. The weight distribution should be in the ratio 70 percent to 30 percent.
- **Step 2:** Lower down your upper body by bending your elbows till your chest is slightly touching the floor. Maintain the weight distribution (70% to 30%) all the time.
- **Step 3:** Return back to the original position, and switch the sides.
- **Step 4:** Perform 10 to 15 repetitions on each side.

Push-ups (Crucifix):

- **Step 1:** Attain the usual push-up position. Place both of your hands wider than shoulder-distance apart. Point your fingers outwards.
- **Step 2:** Lower down your upper body till your chest is slightly touching the floor.
- **Step 3:** Return back to the original position.

- **Step 4:** Perform 10 to 15 repetitions.

Chest Dips:

- **Step 1:** Balance your upper body over a dip bar (you can even use chairs or benches). Raise your entire body by straightening your arms.
- **Step 2:** Lower down your entire body till your elbows attain a perpendicular shape. Lean your upper body forward all through the motion.
- **Step 3:** Return back to the original position.
- **Step 4:** Perform 10 to 15 repetitions.

Diamond Push-ups for chest:

- **Step 1:** Attain a push-up position with your index fingers and thumbs making a diamond shape on the floor.
- **Step 2:** Hold your elbows as near as possible to your sides and bring your upper body down towards the floor till your chest makes contact with your hands on the floor. During the entire motion you need to keep your core muscles, thighs, and glutes tight.
- **Step 3:** Return back to the original position.
- **Step 4:** Perform 12 to 15 repetitions.

4.6) Bodyweight Workouts for Back:

Your back is one of most vital muscle groups which you usually ignore. These muscle groups are used in almost every movement you do during the day, right from bending down to pick something, to moving your rucksack, to putting your baggage on the shelf.

A well-built back and a ripped core work as a team. So, whatever bodyweight workouts you're going to perform will shape up both the muscle groups. In order to develop a strong back, you need to concentrate on your upper back as well as your lower back muscles.

Following are some of the bodyweight exercises for your back:

Sitting Roll-Up:

- **Step 1:** Attain a straight sitting position with straightened legs hip-distance apart. Clip your hands at the back of your head and loosen your feet. Bend your knees a little and tighten your core. Start to lean backward while keeping your legs firm on the floor.
- **Step 2:** Keep on leaning backward till you aren't able to maintain the back straight. Keep your head up and slowly roll through your spine, and gently lower down your entire back on the floor.

- **Step 3:** Start to roll upwards by raising your head, neck, and shoulders using your clipped hands behind your head. Slowly raise your upper body off-the-floor and move your chest forward over your knees.
- **Step 4:** Return back to the original position.
- **Step 5:** Perform 12 to 15 repetitions.

Superman Extension:

- **Step 1:** Lie down on the floor over your belly with straightened legs hip-distance apart. Clip your hands at the back of your head and your toes should be pointed outwards. Straighten out your spine and raise your chest up off-the-floor. Your eyes should focus on the floor to prevent neck pain.
- **Step 2:** Raise your legs upwards off-the-floor and extend both of your arms backward towards your feet. During the motion raise your chest a bit higher off-the-floor and compress your shoulder blades simultaneously.
- **Step 3:** Return back to the original position.
- **Step 4:** Perform 12 to 15 repetitions.

Pike Mount:

- **Step 1:** Attain a plank position using your elbows. Tighten your core and lift your hips as high as possible while try to bring your chest and knees slightly closer. Your body should attain a reverse 'V' shape.

- **Step 2:** Lower down your butts back to plank position while bending your left knee to touch your left elbow. Place your left foot back to attain the plank position and again raise your hips as high as possible. Then, switch the sides. Keep your core tight throughout the motion.
- **Step 3:** Perform 12 to 15 repetitions.

Kneeling Raise:

- **Step 1:** Attain a kneeling position with your hands clipped at the rear of your head, your toes should be pointed outwards, and straighten out your back. Your entire body should be straight in line from your head to knees.
- **Step 2:** Bend your upper body forward as if you're bowing. Move your butts back and lower down your chest till it's nearly parallel to the floor.
- **Step 3:** Hold the position for as long as possible and then return back to the original position. You need to keep your back straight all through the movement.
- **Step 4:** Perform 12 to 15 repetitions.

4.7) Bodyweight Workouts for Legs:

The legs are the largest muscles group in your body; therefore, you definitely need to train them hard! However, you certainly don't require any fancy gym equipment to actually build ripped legs. Your own weight together with some serious determination can help to achieve the desired objectives!

Following are some of the bodyweight workouts for strong and ripped legs:

Squat Tuck Leaps:

- **Step 1**: Attain a standing position with your feet hip-distance apart.
- **Step 2**: Squat down as deep as possible.
- **Step 3**: Assume the standing position quickly by leaping upwards, and try to touch your chest with your knees in the process.
- **Step 4**: Perform 15 to 20 repetitions.

Super Side Lunges:

- **Step 1**: Attain a standing straddle pose by stretching your legs as wide as possible. The longer the legs are, the wider the posture ought to be.
- **Step 2**: Lean your upper body towards your one leg and lower down as deep as possible. The ultimate aim must be to make the back portion of your shin touch your thigh. However, you don't need to put too much strain if the aim is not achievable.
- **Step 3**: Tighten your hips as you return back up to the original position. Perform the entire movement with your other leg.
- **Step 4**: Perform 15 to 20 repetitions.

Leap Lunges:

- **Step 1**: Attain a lunge position by bending your one leg forward (the knee should form a perpendicular angle) and bend your other leg behind you.
- **Step 2**: Quickly jump upwards using your back leg, and swiftly switch the leg positions in the mid-air.
- **Step 3**: Finally, land with your other leg as the forward leg.
- **Step 4**: Perform 15 to 20 repetitions.

Squat Leaps:

- **Step 1**: Attain a standing position with your feet shoulder-distance apart.
- **Step 2**: Lower down your body and assume a squat posture. Try to keep your thighs parallel to the ground.
- **Step 3**: Leap upwards as forcibly as you can by stretching your arms up in the air, and again land in the same squat posture.
- **Step 4**: Perform 15 to 20 repetitions.

Long Leaps:

- **Step 1**: Attain a squat position with your feet shoulder-distance apart.
- **Step 2**: Leap forward with full force to cover as much distance as possible.

- **Step 3:** Continue to repeat the forward leaps to achieve maximum benefits.

Switch Leaps:

- **Step 1:** Attain a squat posture with your feet shoulder-distance apart and your arms by your sides.
- **Step 2:** Leap as high as possible by stretching your arms upwards, and then switch the direction of your posture in mid-air.
- **Step 3:** Land again in a squat posture by lowering your arms in the process.
- **Step 4:** Perform 15 to 20 repetitions as fast as possible.

4.8) Bodyweight Workouts for Awesome Thighs:

Super-ripped thighs easily fill out those specially designed jeans in the best possible ways. These even assist you during tough long runs and cycling exercises.

Following are some of the bodyweight workouts for strong and ripped thighs:

Simple Squats:

- **Step 1:** Attain a standing position with your feet shoulder-distance apart. Clip your hands at the back of your head.
- **Step 2:** Bend your knees and assume a sitting position with your hips in the air. Continue to lower down your hips as deep as possible. During the entire movement, push your knees outwards, and maintain your head straight and up.
- **Step 3:** Swiftly move your hips up and return back to the original position.
- **Step 4:** Perform 15 to 20 repetitions.

Pistol (or One-Legged) Squats:

- **Step 1:** Attain a one-legged standing position and straighten out your other leg before you.
- **Step 2:** Lower down your entire body on that one leg as deep as possible. If possible, assume a sitting position and let the back of your shin touch your thighs.
- **Step 3:** Slowly return back to the standing position. Then, switch the sides and perform the squat with your other leg.
- **Step 4:** Perform 10 to 15 repetitions.

4.9) Bodyweight Workouts for Calves:

Calf muscles are one of the toughest to develop, especially for those with smaller calves. Because these muscles are found in the lower part of the legs, some additional size there forms the illusion that your entire leg is lot bigger. Well-built calves are accompanied by the extra advantage of enhanced athleticism. It takes a lot of strength out of your calves in order to perform high jumps or sprint explosively.

Following are some of the bodyweight workouts for strong and ripped Calves:

Calf Stretch against Wall:

- **Step 1:** Attain a standing position against a wall by placing both of your hands on it and maintain a distance of quite a few feet in between your legs and the wall. Gently place your one foot forward.
- **Step 2:** Lean your entire upper body towards the wall. Maintain your head, butts and back heel straight in line.
- **Step 3:** Try to press your heel into the floor, and hold the position for 20 to 25 seconds. After that, switch the sides.
- **Step 4:** Perform 10 to 15 repetitions.

Foam Roll Calves:

- **Step 1:** Attain a sitting position on the floor. Gently place a foam roller below one of your legs. Cross over your other leg over that leg or you can even place it on the floor to offer some support.

- **Step 2:** Firmly place both of your hands behind you or at your sides, and press them down to lift your butts up off-the-floor. This move will put a lot of your weight on your calves. Roll over the foam roller from below your knee up to your ankle. Halt at the points where your feel strain for 15 to 25 seconds. After that, switch the sides.
- **Step 3:** Perform 10 to 15 repetitions.

Standing Calf raise:

Note: For this particular workout, you'll require a step or a block to stand on, and something to hold on to maintain your balance.

- **Step 1:** Stand straight on a step or a block with your feet on its edge and lower down your heels as deep as you can.
- **Step 2:** Gently lift your heels up as high as you can. Hold the position for some time, and then gently lower down your heels again as deep as you can.
- **Step 3:** Don't halt the movement at the bottom, and instantly begin the next motion.
- **Step 4:** Perform 15 to 20 repetitions.

Lunge Pulses:

- **Step 1**: Attain a standing position and hold a broomstick in your hands over your head, and keep your feet hip-distance apart.
- **Step 2**: Place your one foot forward to attain a lunge position. Your front knee should form 90 degrees angle. Bend the knee of the other leg behind you.
- **Step 3**: Hold this position and pulse up by lifting your back leg knee. Then, pulse down by lowering your back leg knee to finish one pulse. Perform up to 20 pulses, and then switch the sides.
- **Step 4**: Perform 15 to 20 repetitions.

****

These were some of the vital bodyweight exercises for your entire body.

Conclusion

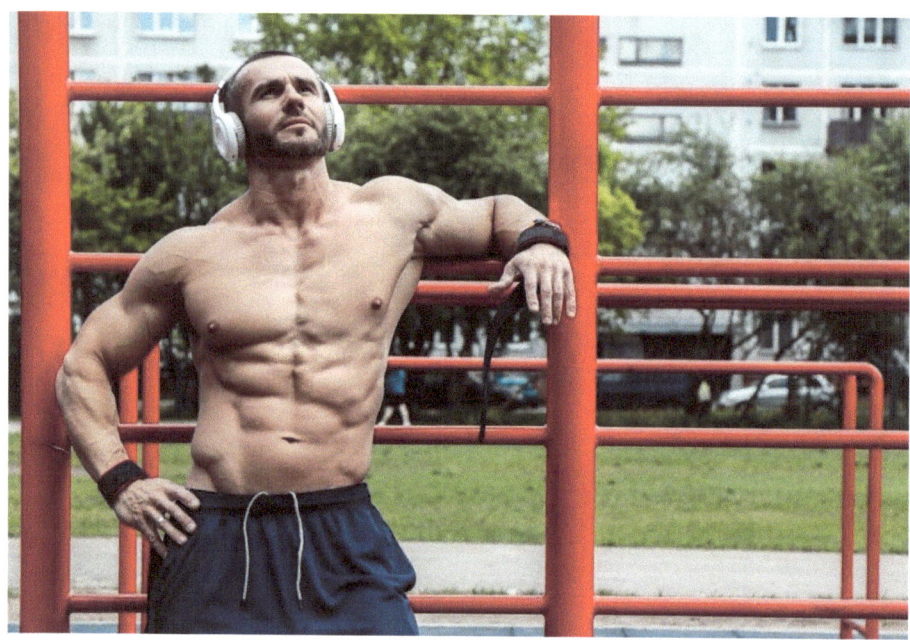

Besides the notable levels of stamina that can be developed, bodyweight exercises for your overall body need brilliant body and mind control. Body maneuvers in the air enhance response through the cerebral system, mechanoreceptors as well as various other neural features, which when pooled together possibly gives a properly planned bodyweight training a significant advantage over free weight training, in terms of stamina and muscles development.

As bodyweight strength output depends on various factors, for instance, limb lengths, the cross-sectional region of the muscle groups, the angle of pressure on various joints, and several other neural features, building all these features speedily along with body mass and stamina will assist you in achieving fast and amazing results.

Anybody who has gone through both bodyweight training, as well as weight training sessions, would surely attest strongly in favor of bodyweight training. The fundamental fact is that force-is-force! Therefore, if you can put the appropriate amount of pressure on the designated muscles via various bodyweight workouts, you'll definitely feel an amazing increase in both body mass and stamina. Bodyweight exercises will offer you structured developments via which the impulse on the designated muscles can be enhanced without gaining body mass.

Bodyweight training skill development is relatively different from free-weight training. They follow entirely diverse zones. Their levels of development are divided by the capability in any prior skill progression along with stamina development. This intricacy of skill developments, as well as the unreliable nature of various individuals and their eventual objectives, makes bodyweight training and free weight training - an entirely different league.

One of the huge dilemmas which many individuals come across with bodyweight training is that it's quite difficult to witness fast results which is very much in contrast to the free weight training where you can put more weight on the bar each session. But you always need to bear in mind that the key to success here is enormous willpower and consistency which is quite similar to any other sports training. You'll surely achieve maximum benefits if you practice consistently and hard! That's guaranteed! This is applicable to any kind of program whether bodyweight, or free weight or any other type of physical training.

For those individuals who desire to do a mixture of bodyweight and free weight exercises, you can feel all by yourself that a lot of weight training workouts are pretty much related to pushing and pulling workouts. You can substitute some of these bodyweight workouts with your weight training exercises.

There's absolutely no restriction on how much strength you can gain by just utilizing your own bodyweight during workouts. The key trick is to know all about how to fully and efficiently control your body movements to achieve maximum benefits.

You can assess your audacity against some of these bodyweight moves and check how many you're actually able to carry out! Huge surprises might be in store for you when you come to know about the feats which presently you're able to achieve! With consistent practice and strong willpower, those bodyweight movements which appeared impossible on your initial attempt can definitely be performed and subdued.

Bodyweight workouts can be performed by anyone and anywhere! It's certainly good news for all those individuals who don't have any access to free weights or a gym, or who desire to exercise more frequently, or just wish a drastic change in their daily workout routine. It's also great for your joints!

Bear in mind that if you're not able to do some of the basic bodyweight workouts for more than 15 seconds, then you're strongly advised not to perform the similar fundamental move with any free weight equipment. For instance, if you're not able to perform 20 push-ups then there's no reason for you to perform heavyweight bench presses. The prime reason is that for bodyweight workouts, 15 seconds though might be a good start but is not at all the final limit, particularly when your ultimate objective should be to achieve advanced levels of anaerobic stamina.

You must try to perform all the bodyweight workouts as described in this book. After you accomplish the basic objectives for each bodyweight workout, you can then move on to weight training. You'll be surely astonished how swiftly you'll improve your snatch, deadlift, or any other weight training routine.

This book has genuinely touched as well as explained various vital topics including the needs and benefits of bodyweight exercises. The book has also shared with you various in-depth details about bodyweight equipment, diet and nutrition, and rest and recovery. The book has thoroughly revealed all the warm-up and stretching routines which should be performed before starting your workouts, and all the bodyweight exercises which cover nearly your entire body parts such as arms, neck, and shoulders, core muscles, chest region, the back region, legs, thighs, calves, etc.

And this brings our book to an end! We sincerely believe that this book will immensely assist you to perform all the detailed bodyweight exercises with full confidence and ease, and also help you to achieve superior physical ability, and a grand flattering ripped body with **GREAT SUCESS!**

Thanks again for downloading this book! And if you've really enjoyed reading this book, then I'd like to ask you for a favor! Would you please like to leave a review for this book? It'd be deeply appreciated!